THE RESILIENT MINDSET

BOOST PERFORMANCE, STRENGTHEN MENTAL TOUGHNESS, ENHANCE EMOTIONAL STABILITY, AND UNLOCK YOUR LIMITLESS POTENTIAL

PREM SAGAR SUNCHU

YOUR FREE GIFT !!

As a token of my thanks for taking out time to read my book, I would like to offer you a **Free-Gift**:

Click the Below Link and Download your **Free eBook PDF**.

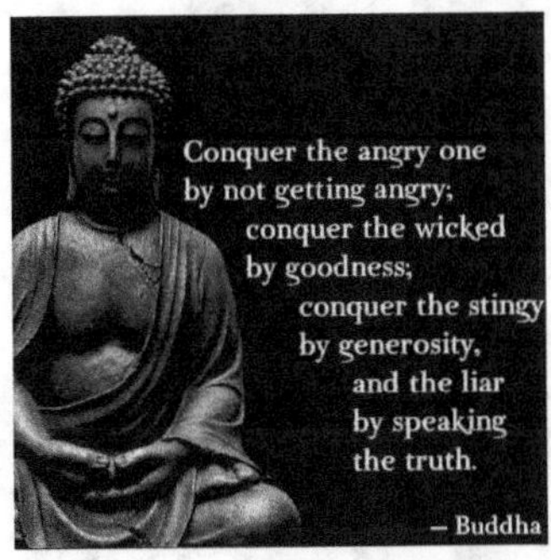

"The Power of Community: Thriving Together"

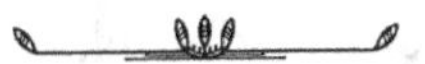

ABOUT THE AUTHOR

Prem Sagar Sunchu, the Accomplished Author of "The Resilient Mindset"

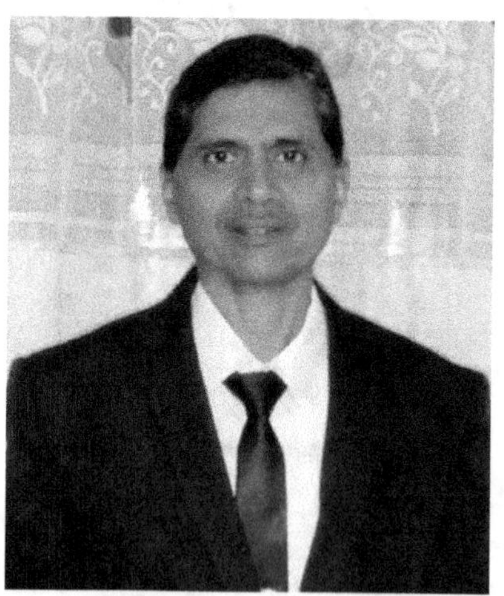

Meet Mr. Prem Sagar, an ordinary soul born in the vibrant city of Secunderabad, India, where the tapestry of life weaves stories of resilience and dreams. His journey is a testament to the power of perpetual learning, where every encounter is a lesson, and every moment holds the potential for growth.

A man of many dimensions, Mr. Sagar embodies the qualities of a perpetual student, a dedicated listener, and a dreamer who gazes at the stars but keeps his feet firmly grounded. His aspirations soar high, and his relentless pursuit of them is fueled by a genuine desire to make a positive impact on those around him.

Having served as a Chief Manager in the prestigious State Bank of India, Mr. Sagar brings a wealth of experience from the world of banking. However, for him, retirement isn't a conclusion but a commencement—a reminder that life's true journey begins when one can reflect on the wisdom gained from the first innings.

In Mr. Sagar's view, retirement is not a retreat but a stepping stone to a realm of infinite possibilities. It's an opportunity to surpass the ordinary, where the canvas of life awaits new brushstrokes of creativity and purpose. For him, the "be good and do good policy" isn't just a mantra; it's a guiding principle that shapes his approach to life.

As he embraces the second innings, Mr. Sagar encourages others to view retirement not as a winding down but as a springboard to new endeavors. It's a time when accumulated wisdom meets fresh energy, and the monotony of routine gives way to the vibrancy of creativity. His belief is clear: retirement is not just a number; it's a chapter where the richness of experience meets the possibilities in abundance.

In the world of Mr. Prem Sagar, retirement is not a period of rest but a canvas waiting to be painted with the colors of newfound wisdom, creativity, and a different outlook on life.

Prem Sagar Sunchu
M.Com, LLM, Certified Independent Director (IICA) GOI, Author, Sole Arbitrator and Legal Consultant, Freelancer

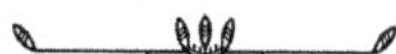

ACKNOWLEDGEMENTS

In profound gratitude, I extend heartfelt appreciation to my amazing parents. To my caring and resilient mother, **Smt. S.L. Lakshmi**, who gracefully navigated the challenges of my father's service transfers, made countless sacrifices to bind our family together. My father, **Shri S.R. Lakshman Rao**, stands as my enduring role model—his post-retirement vibrancy, marked by a dedicated hobby of reading and writing, serves as the very foundation that propels me into the realm of authorship. A debt of gratitude is owed to my beautiful wife, **Smt. S.P. Padma Sree** is a constant source of inspiration, unwavering strength, and invaluable guidance. Balancing family responsibilities and the intricate path of an author, her presence has been the foundation of my journey.

To my handsome sons, **S.P. Gautam Sagar**, **S.P. Prayag Sagar**, and **S.P. Akshaj Sagar**, whose unwavering support and responsibility bear testament to the great strength they provide. Their motivation fuels my endeavors across all the diverse traits I undertake.

I owe thanks to **Mr. Som Bathla**, an **Amazon #1 Bestselling** author, for his mentorship, motivation, and guidance in the realms of

Writing, Self-Publishing, and Launching Books. His support has been instrumental in initiating my journey as an Authorpreneur.

My Sincere thanks to **Mr. Sooraj Achar**, who is also an Amazon Bestselling Author, for his **Professional Editing,** Formatting, and Publishing support.

In acknowledging these pillars of support, I am reminded that the tapestry of my life and authorial pursuit is woven with threads of love, sacrifice, and inspiration. With profound thanks to my family, who stand as my bedrock of strength and motivation.

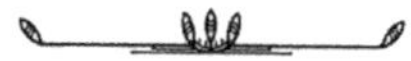

DEDICATION

To the guiding stars of my universe—my Parents, Grandparents, Parents-in-law, Brothers, Sisters, the cherished members of our extended Family and Friends. Their unwavering support and boundless encouragement have been the driving force behind my Author Journey.

In the tapestry of my life, each of them has woven threads of inspiration and resilience, transforming mere words into stories and dreams into realities. Their confidence in me has been a constant source of strength, propelling me forward through the path of this journey.

With heartfelt gratitude, I dedicate the pages of my work to the pillars of love and encouragement that they are, recognizing that every word I pen is a tribute to the collective spirit of our family. May this dedication reflect the depth of my appreciation for the profound impact they have had on my creative journey.

"The Resilient Mindset" is my second book in the series of five books-**"The Resilient Mind."**

CONTENTS

INTRODUCTION

"Resilience is not about overcoming; it's about becoming." – Sherri Mandell

In a world filled with constant change, challenges, and uncertainties, the ability to bounce back from adversity and thrive amidst difficulties is more critical than ever. This book, "The Resilient Mindset," is your guide to cultivating the strength, adaptability, and positive habits necessary to not just survive but truly thrive in life.

Understanding Resilience

Resilience is often misunderstood as a trait that only a few possess, but research shows that it is a skill that anyone can develop. In Chapter 1, we explore what resilience truly means, its psychological and neurological underpinnings, and its profound benefits. We also provide tools to assess your current resilience level, setting the foundation for growth and improvement.

Building a Resilient Foundation

A resilient mindset starts with a solid foundation. Chapter 2 delves into developing self-awareness, embracing a growth mindset, strengthening emotional intelligence, and setting and achieving goals. By understanding your triggers, cultivating mindfulness, and fostering a mindset open to growth, you can build the robust mental framework needed to face life's challenges head-on.

Overcoming Adversity

Challenges and failures are inevitable, but they can be powerful catalysts for growth. Chapter 3 provides strategies for coping with life's difficulties, learning from failures, managing stress and anxiety, and navigating grief and loss. Through real-life case studies and scientific research, this chapter shows how overcoming adversity can lead to personal transformation and resilience.

Cultivating Positive Habits

Daily habits play a crucial role in maintaining resilience. Chapter 4 highlights the power of routines, the importance of physical health, the role of quality sleep, and the benefits of practicing gratitude and optimism. By incorporating these positive habits into your life, you can create a strong foundation for sustained mental and emotional well-being.

Strengthening Relationships

Strong social connections are a cornerstone of resilience. Chapter 5 explores building a support network, effective communication skills, collaborative problem-solving, and supporting others in their resilience journey. Meaningful relationships provide the support and encouragement needed to navigate challenges and celebrate successes.

Thriving in Life

Ultimately, resilience is about thriving, not just surviving. Chapter 6 focuses on embracing change and uncertainty, finding purpose and meaning, sustaining long-term resilience, and celebrating progress. By embracing adaptability, discovering your passions, and continuously improving, you can lead a fulfilling and resilient life.

Your Journey to a Resilient Mindset

"The Resilient Mindset" is more than just a book; it is a comprehensive guide to transforming your life through resilience. Each chapter is designed to provide you with practical insights, actionable strategies, and inspiring stories to help you build and maintain a resilient mindset. Whether you are facing personal challenges, professional setbacks, or simply seeking to improve your overall well-being, this book offers the tools and knowledge you need to thrive.

As you embark on this journey, remember that resilience is not a destination but a continuous process of growth and adaptation. By committing to developing a resilient mindset, you are taking a powerful step toward a more fulfilling, balanced, and successful life. Welcome to "The Resilient Mindset" – your path to thriving in every aspect of your life.

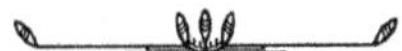

MAY I ASK YOU FOR A SMALL FAVOR?

I want to express my sincere gratitude for choosing to invest your time in reading this book. Your decision to explore this work among countless others means a lot to me.

I hope that within these pages, you've discovered actionable insights that can enhance your daily life. Your journey doesn't have to end here, though.

May I kindly request an additional 30 seconds of your valuable time?

Sharing your thoughts about the book through a review would be immensely appreciated. Your review serves as a beacon, guiding other readers to take a chance on my books. It's a small gesture that carries significant weight in the world of authors.

To submit your review effortlessly, please click on the link below. It will take you directly to the book's review page:

"The Resilient Mindset"

Alternatively, you can also find the **"Reviews Section"** of this book's page on Amazon.

Your review will require just a minute of your time but will make a monumental difference in helping me connect with a broader audience and I eagerly look forward to reading your review.

Once again, thank you for your unwavering support of my work.

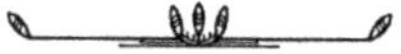

DISCLAIMER

This book is for educational purposes only. Readers acknowledge that the author does not render legal, financial, medical, or professional advice. The content within this book has been derived from various sources. Please consult a licensed professional before attempting any techniques outlined in this book.

By reading this document, the reader agrees that under no circumstances is the author responsible for any direct or indirect losses incurred as a result of the use of the information contained within this document, including but not limited to errors, omissions, or inaccuracies.

Adherence to all applicable laws and regulations, including international, federal, state, and local governing professional licensing, business practices, advertising, and all other jurisdictions, is the sole responsibility of the purchaser or reader.

Neither the author nor the publisher assumes any responsibility or liability whatsoever on behalf of the purchaser or reader of these materials. Any perceived slight of any individual or organization is purely unintentional.

CHAPTER 1

UNDERSTANDING RESILIENCE

"Resilience is not about avoiding the storm but learning to dance in the rain." – Unknown

Introduction

Resilience is the remarkable capacity to recover from difficulties and adapt to challenging circumstances. It's more than just bouncing back—it's about thriving despite adversity. Understanding resilience can transform our approach to life's inevitable ups and downs, fostering a mindset that embraces challenges as opportunities for growth.

1.1 The Definition of Resilience

What is Resilience?

Resilience is the ability to withstand, adapt to, and recover from stress and adversity. It involves maintaining or quickly regaining mental health during and after experiencing life stressors. This trait is not an innate quality but a set of behaviors, thoughts, and actions that can be learned and developed by anyone.

The Importance of Mental Fortitude

Mental fortitude is the backbone of resilience. It allows individuals to face adversity head-on, without succumbing to stress or negative emotions. Those with strong mental fortitude can navigate life's challenges more effectively, maintaining their composure and focus even under pressure. This strength helps in overcoming obstacles and pursuing long-term goals, contributing to overall well-being and success.

1.2 The Science Behind Resilience

Psychological and Neurological Basis

Research has shown that resilience is rooted in both psychological and neurological processes. Psychologically, it involves traits like optimism, emotional regulation, and the ability to reframe negative experiences. Neurologically, resilience is linked to the brain's ability to adapt through neuroplasticity, which allows the brain to form new connections and pathways in response to experiences and learning.

The Role of Neuroplasticity

Neuroplasticity is the brain's ability to reorganize itself by forming new neural connections. This adaptability is crucial for resilience, as it enables individuals to learn from experiences and adapt to new situations. Studies have shown that engaging in activities that promote neuroplasticity, such as mindfulness meditation, physical exercise, and continuous learning, can enhance resilience.

1.3 The Benefits of a Resilient Mindset

Enhanced Emotional Well-being

A resilient mindset contributes significantly to emotional well-being. Resilient individuals tend to experience lower levels of depression and anxiety. They are better equipped to handle stress and recover from emotional setbacks. This emotional stability promotes a positive outlook on life, even in the face of challenges.

Better Stress Management

Resilience plays a critical role in stress management. Those with a resilient mindset can maintain calmness and clarity during stressful situations. They are more likely to employ effective coping strategies, such as problem-solving, seeking social support, and engaging in healthy activities, which mitigate the adverse effects of stress.

1.4 Assessing Your Current Resilience Level

Understanding your current resilience level is the first step towards building a stronger, more resilient mindset. Self-reflection exercises can help identify areas where resilience is already strong and areas that need improvement.

Self-Reflection Exercises

1. **Identify Past Challenges:** Reflect on past difficulties and how you responded. What strategies did you use to cope? What did you learn from these experiences?

2. **Recognize Strengths and Weaknesses:** Assess your strengths and areas for growth. Are there patterns in your responses to stress? Understanding these can guide your resilience-building efforts.

Resilience Self-Assessment Tools

Several self-assessment tools can provide insights into your resilience level. These tools typically involve questionnaires that measure various aspects of resilience, such as emotional regulation, optimism, and social support. Utilizing these tools can help create a personalized plan for enhancing resilience.

Case Studies

Case Study 1: Overcoming Personal Loss

Jane, a successful businesswoman, faced the tragic loss of her spouse. Initially, she struggled with profound grief and depression. However, through therapy, support from friends, and engaging in activities that promoted her mental health, Jane gradually rebuilt her life. She started a foundation in her spouse's memory, which gave her a renewed sense of purpose and helped her cope with her loss. Jane's story illustrates the power of resilience in overcoming personal tragedy.

Case Study 2: Thriving After Professional Setback

Mark, an aspiring entrepreneur, faced a significant setback when his startup failed. Devastated but determined, Mark sought mentorship and invested time in learning from his mistakes. He adopted a growth mindset and focused on personal development. Eventually, he launched a new, successful venture. Mark's journey demonstrates how resilience can turn failure into a stepping stone for future success.

Conclusion

Resilience is a vital quality that can be nurtured and developed. By understanding its definition, scientific basis, and benefits, and by assessing and actively working on our resilience levels, we can better navigate life's challenges. Cultivating resilience not only enhances our emotional well-being but also equips us with the tools to manage stress and grow from adversity.

Resources

1. **Books**

- "The Resilience Factor" by Karen Reivich and Andrew Shatté

- "Resilience: The Science of Mastering Life's Greatest Challenges" by Steven Southwick and Dennis Charney

2. **Articles**

- "The Neuroscience of Resilience" - Harvard Business Review

- "Building Your Resilience" - American Psychological Association

3. **Websites**

- American Psychological Association (www.apa.org)

- Greater Good Science Center (www.greatergood.berkeley.edu)

By incorporating these resources and insights, you can embark on a journey to cultivate a resilient mindset and transform your approach to life's challenges.

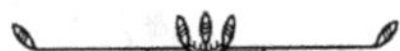

CHAPTER 2

BUILDING A RESILIENT FOUNDATION

*"Strength does not come from physical capacity.
It comes from an indomitable will." – Mahatma
Gandhi*

Introduction

A resilient foundation is crucial for weathering life's storms. It equips us with the tools to bounce back from setbacks, adapt to changes, and keep moving forward. Building this foundation involves developing self-awareness, embracing a growth mindset, strengthening emotional intelligence, and setting and achieving goals. Each of these components contributes to a more resilient, adaptable, and fulfilled life.

2.1 Developing Self-Awareness

Understanding Your Triggers

Self-awareness is the cornerstone of resilience. It involves understanding your emotions, thoughts, and behaviors, especially in stressful situations. Recognizing what triggers your stress or anxiety can help you manage your reactions more effectively. Start by keeping a journal to note down moments of intense emotion and the circumstances surrounding them. Over time, patterns will emerge, revealing your specific triggers.

Cultivating Mindfulness

Mindfulness is a powerful tool for enhancing self-awareness. It involves paying attention to the present moment without judgment. Regular mindfulness practice, such as meditation or mindful breathing, can increase your awareness of thoughts and feelings, making it easier to manage them. Research shows that mindfulness can reduce stress, improve focus, and increase emotional regulation.

2.2 Embracing a Growth Mindset

Fixed vs. Growth Mindset

A growth mindset is the belief that abilities and intelligence can be developed through dedication and hard work. This contrasts with a fixed mindset, where individuals believe their qualities are set in stone. Embracing a growth mindset fosters resilience by encouraging perseverance, learning from failures, and seeing challenges as opportunities.

Strategies to Foster Growth

To cultivate a growth mindset, start by reframing challenges as opportunities to learn. When faced with a setback, ask yourself what you can learn from the experience. Surround yourself with supportive people who encourage growth and provide constructive feedback. Finally, celebrate your efforts and progress, not just the end results.

2.3 Strengthening Emotional Intelligence

Recognizing and Managing Emotions

Emotional intelligence (EI) is the ability to recognize, understand, and manage our own emotions and those of others. High EI is linked to better stress management, improved relationships, and greater resilience. Start by labeling your emotions accurately. Instead of saying "I feel bad," try to pinpoint the exact emotion, such as "I feel frustrated" or "I feel anxious." This clarity helps in addressing the underlying issues more effectively.

Building Empathy and Social Skills

Empathy, a key component of EI, involves understanding and sharing the feelings of others. It enhances social connections and builds support networks, which are vital for resilience. Practice active listening, which involves fully focusing on the speaker, understanding their message, responding thoughtfully, and withholding judgment. Improving your social skills through better communication, conflict resolution, and collaboration can also enhance your resilience.

2.4 Setting and Achieving Goals

SMART Goals Framework

Setting clear, achievable goals gives direction and purpose, enhancing resilience. The SMART framework is a useful tool for goal setting. Ensure your goals are Specific, Measurable, Achievable, Relevant, and Time-bound. For example, instead of saying, "I want to be healthier," a SMART goal would be, "I will exercise for 30 minutes, five times a week, for the next three months."

The Power of Small Wins

Small wins create a sense of progress and achievement, boosting motivation and resilience. Break down your larger goals into smaller, manageable tasks. Celebrate these small victories to maintain momentum and build confidence. Research indicates that recognizing and celebrating small achievements can significantly enhance overall motivation and well-being.

Case Studies

Case Study 1: Developing Self-Awareness and Mindfulness

Jane, a high school teacher, struggled with overwhelming stress due to her demanding job and personal life. By keeping a journal, she identified her primary stressors and began practicing mindfulness meditation. Within a few months, Jane reported a significant decrease in stress levels and an improved ability to handle challenging situations calmly. Her journey illustrates how self-awareness and mindfulness can build a resilient foundation.

Case Study 2: Embracing a Growth Mindset and Setting Goals

Tom, an aspiring entrepreneur, faced numerous failures in his early ventures. Instead of giving up, he adopted a growth mindset, viewing each failure as a learning opportunity. He set SMART goals for his next project, focusing on achievable milestones. By celebrating small wins and learning from setbacks, Tom eventually built a successful business. His story demonstrates the power of a growth mindset and goal setting in building resilience.

Conclusion

Building a resilient foundation is an ongoing process that involves self-awareness, a growth mindset, emotional intelligence, and effective goal setting. These elements interconnect to create a robust framework for handling life's challenges with strength and adaptability. By developing these skills, we can enhance our ability to bounce back from setbacks and thrive in the face of adversity.

Resources

1. **Books**

   - "Mindset: The New Psychology of Success" by Carol S. Dweck

   - "Emotional Intelligence 2.0" by Travis Bradberry and Jean Greaves

2. **Articles**

   - "The Science of Mindfulness" – Harvard Health Publishing

   - "Emotional Intelligence: Why It Can Matter More Than IQ" – Daniel Goleman

3. **Websites**

- ○ Greater Good Science Center (www.greatergood.ber keley.edu)

- ○ Mindful (www.mindful.org)

4. Self-Assessment Tools

- ○ Mindfulness-Based Stress Reduction (MBSR) programs

- ○ Emotional Intelligence Appraisal tests

CHAPTER 3

OVERCOMING ADVERSITY

"The human capacity for burden is like bamboo—far more flexible than you'd ever believe at first glance." – Jodi Picoult

Introduction

Life inevitably presents us with challenges, failures, stress, and loss. How we respond to these adversities shapes our resilience and our ability to thrive despite them. Overcoming adversity involves effective problem-solving, emotional regulation, learning from failure, managing stress, and navigating through grief and loss. This chapter explores practical strategies and inspiring stories that illustrate how resilience can be built and strengthened in the face of life's toughest moments.

3.1 Coping with Life's Challenges

Techniques for Problem-Solving

Effective problem-solving is a crucial skill for overcoming adversity. Start by clearly defining the problem. Break it down into manageable parts and brainstorm possible solutions. Evaluate the pros and cons of each solution and choose the most feasible one. Implement the solution and assess its effectiveness. If it doesn't work, revisit your options and try another approach. This iterative process helps build resilience by fostering a proactive attitude towards challenges.

Strategies for Emotional Regulation

Emotional regulation is the ability to manage and respond to emotional experiences in a healthy way. Techniques such as deep breathing, mindfulness meditation, and cognitive reframing can help. Deep breathing activates the parasympathetic nervous system, reducing stress and anxiety. Mindfulness meditation increases awareness and acceptance of emotions. Cognitive reframing involves changing the way we interpret and respond to situations, helping us view challenges from a more balanced perspective.

3.2 Learning from Failure

The Value of Mistakes

Failure is an inevitable part of life and a powerful teacher. Mistakes offer valuable insights and opportunities for growth. By analyzing failures, we can identify what went wrong and how to improve. This process fosters a growth mindset, which is essential for resilience. Embracing failure as a learning experience rather than a setback can lead to greater innovation, creativity, and success.

Building a Failure-Resilient Attitude

Developing a failure-resilient attitude involves changing our perception of failure. Instead of viewing it as a reflection of our abilities, see it as a necessary step towards growth. Celebrate efforts and progress rather than just the outcomes. Surround yourself with supportive people who encourage a positive perspective on failure. This attitude not only enhances resilience but also promotes a lifelong love of learning and personal development.

3.3 Managing Stress and Anxiety

Effective Stress-Reduction Techniques

Managing stress is vital for maintaining resilience. Effective techniques include physical activity, relaxation exercises, and time management. Regular physical activity releases endorphins, which improve mood and reduce stress. Relaxation exercises such as progressive muscle relaxation and guided imagery can help calm the mind and body. Time management techniques like prioritizing tasks and setting realistic goals reduce the feeling of being overwhelmed.

Building a Stress-Resilient Mindset

A stress-resilient mindset involves viewing stress as a challenge rather than a threat. This perspective can be developed through cognitive-behavioral strategies such as positive self-talk and realistic thinking. Positive self-talk involves replacing negative thoughts with positive affirmations. Realistic thinking focuses on evaluating situations objectively and identifying practical solutions. This mindset not only reduces stress but also enhances overall resilience.

3.4 Navigating Through Grief and Loss

Understanding the Grieving Process

Grief is a natural response to loss and involves a range of emotions, including sadness, anger, and confusion. Understanding the grieving process can help us navigate through it more effectively. The stages of grief—denial, anger, bargaining, depression, and acceptance—are not linear and can vary greatly among individuals. Allowing yourself to experience these emotions without judgment is crucial for healing.

Building Strength Through Adversity

Grief, though painful, can also be a source of strength. Finding meaning in loss, whether through personal growth or helping others, can transform grief into a source of resilience. Support from friends, family, or support groups can provide comfort and understanding. Engaging in self-care activities, such as journaling, exercise, and creative expression, can also aid in the healing process.

Case Studies

Case Study 1: Coping with Life's Challenges

Maria, a single mother, faced significant financial and emotional challenges after losing her job. Through problem-solving techniques, she identified ways to cut expenses and sought out new job opportunities. She also practiced mindfulness and deep breathing exercises to manage her anxiety. Maria's resilience grew as she navigated these challenges, ultimately finding a better job and achieving greater financial stability.

Case Study 2: Learning from Failure and Managing Stress

David, an ambitious entrepreneur, faced a major setback when his startup failed. Instead of giving up, he analyzed his mistakes and sought feedback from mentors. He adopted a growth mindset, viewing his failure as a learning opportunity. David also implemented stress-reduction techniques like regular exercise and time management. His resilience paid off when he successfully launched a new venture, applying the lessons he learned from his past failure.

Conclusion

Overcoming adversity is an integral part of building resilience. By developing effective problem-solving skills, emotional regulation, a positive attitude towards failure, and stress management techniques, we can navigate life's challenges with greater ease. Understanding and embracing the grieving process further strengthens our ability to overcome loss and find meaning in adversity. These skills and perspectives not only enhance our resilience but also enrich our lives, enabling us to thrive despite difficulties.

Resources

1. **Books**

    ○ "The Obstacle Is the Way: The Timeless Art of Turning Trials into Triumph" by Ryan Holiday

    ○ "Option B: Facing Adversity, Building Resilience, and Finding Joy" by Sheryl Sandberg and Adam Grant

2. **Articles**

    ○ "The Science of Resilience" – American Psychological Association

    ○ "How to Turn a Stressful Situation Into a Positive One" – Harvard Business Review

3. Websites

- American Psychological Association (www.apa.org)

- National Institute of Mental Health (www.nimh.nih.gov)

4. Support Groups

- GriefShare (www.griefshare.org)

- Anxiety and Depression Association of America (www.adaa.org)

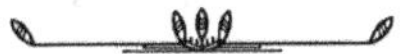

CHAPTER 4

CULTIVATING POSITIVE HABITS

"We are what we repeatedly do. Excellence, then, is not an act, but a habit." – Aristotle

Introduction

Building resilience is an ongoing process that benefits greatly from cultivating positive habits. These habits form the foundation of our daily lives, influencing our mental, physical, and emotional well-being. Establishing a routine, maintaining physical health, ensuring quality sleep, and practicing gratitude and optimism are essential components of a resilient lifestyle. This chapter explores the power of these habits and how they contribute to building a stronger, more adaptable self.

4.1 The Power of Routine

Building Daily Habits for Resilience

Routine provides structure and predictability, which are key elements in fostering resilience. By establishing daily habits, we create a sense of stability and control, even in the face of uncertainty. Start by identifying small, manageable habits that align with your goals. Consistency is crucial; the more you practice these habits, the more ingrained they become. For example, setting aside time each day for mindfulness or exercise can significantly enhance your resilience.

Morning and Evening Rituals

Morning and evening rituals set the tone for your day and prepare your mind for rest, respectively. Morning rituals might include activities like meditation, exercise, or journaling, which can boost your mood and energy levels. Evening rituals, such as reading or practicing gratitude, help you unwind and reflect on the day. These rituals not only enhance your well-being but also create a sense of routine that supports resilience.

4.2 Physical Health and Resilience

Exercise and Mental Strength

Physical activity is a powerful tool for building mental resilience. Regular exercise releases endorphins, which improve mood and reduce stress. It also enhances cognitive function, increases energy levels, and promotes better sleep. Whether it's a daily walk, yoga, or a more intense workout, incorporating physical activity into your routine can have profound effects on your mental and emotional health.

The Role of Nutrition in Mental Well-being

Nutrition plays a vital role in supporting mental well-being. A balanced diet rich in fruits, vegetables, whole grains, and lean proteins provides the nutrients your brain needs to function optimally. Omega-3 fatty acids, found in fish and flaxseed, have been shown to improve mood and cognitive function. Staying hydrated and reducing the intake of processed foods and sugars can also enhance your mental resilience.

4.3 Sleep and Recovery

The Importance of Quality Sleep

Quality sleep is crucial for resilience. It allows your body and mind to recover and rejuvenate. Lack of sleep impairs cognitive function, increases stress levels, and weakens the immune system. Aim for 7-9 hours of sleep each night to ensure you are well-rested and capable of handling daily challenges effectively.

Techniques for Better Sleep Hygiene

Improving sleep hygiene can help you achieve better quality sleep. Establish a regular sleep schedule by going to bed and waking up at the same time each day. Create a restful environment by keeping your bedroom cool, dark, and quiet. Avoid caffeine and electronics before bedtime, and engage in relaxing activities such as reading or taking a warm bath. These practices promote better sleep and enhance overall resilience.

4.4 Practicing Gratitude and Optimism

The Benefits of a Positive Outlook

A positive outlook can significantly enhance resilience. Practicing gratitude and optimism shifts your focus from negative to positive aspects of life, fostering a sense of well-being and hope. Research has shown that individuals who regularly practice gratitude experience lower stress levels, better physical health, and improved relationships.

Daily Practices for Gratitude

Incorporate gratitude into your daily routine by keeping a gratitude journal. Each day, write down three things you are grateful for. This practice helps you focus on positive experiences and fosters a more optimistic outlook. Additionally, expressing gratitude to others, whether through a note, a call, or a simple thank you, can strengthen your social connections and enhance your resilience.

Case Studies

Case Study 1: The Power of Routine

Samantha, a nurse working in a high-stress environment, found herself overwhelmed by anxiety and burnout. She decided to establish a morning routine that included 15 minutes of meditation, a healthy breakfast, and a short walk. In the evening, she practiced gratitude by writing in her journal. These simple routines provided her with a sense of control and stability, significantly reducing her stress and increasing her resilience over time.

Case Study 2: Physical Health and Sleep

John, a software developer, struggled with insomnia and chronic stress due to his demanding job. He started incorporating regular exercise into his schedule, focusing on cardiovascular workouts and strength training. He also improved his sleep hygiene by setting a regular bedtime, reducing screen time before bed, and creating a relaxing bedtime ritual. These changes not only improved his sleep quality but also enhanced his overall mental and physical resilience.

Conclusion

Cultivating positive habits is essential for building and maintaining resilience. By establishing a routine, prioritizing physical health, ensuring quality sleep, and practicing gratitude and optimism, we create a solid foundation for navigating life's challenges. These habits, when practiced consistently, enhance our ability to adapt, recover, and thrive in the face of adversity.

Resources

1. **Books**

- "Atomic Habits: An Easy & Proven Way to Build Good Habits & Break Bad Ones" by James Clear

- "The Miracle Morning: The Not-So-Obvious Secret Guaranteed to Transform Your Life (Before 8AM)" by Hal Elrod

2. **Articles**

- "The Importance of Routines" – Psychology Today

- "The Benefits of Physical Activity" – Centers for Disease Control and Prevention

3. **Websites**

- National Sleep Foundation (www.sleepfoundation.org)

- Positive Psychology (www.positivepsychology.com)

4. **Apps**

- Headspace (for meditation and mindfulness)

- MyFitnessPal (for tracking nutrition and exercise)

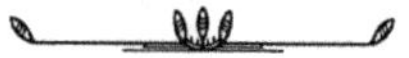

CHAPTER 5

STRENGTHENING RELATIONSHIPS

"Connection is the energy that is created between people when they feel seen, heard, and valued." – Brené Brown

Introduction

Our relationships form the bedrock of our resilience. They provide us with support, encouragement, and a sense of belonging. Strengthening these relationships is crucial not only for our well-being but also for the well-being of those around us. This chapter explores how to build a supportive network, develop effective communication skills, engage in collaborative problem-solving, and support others in their resilience journey.

5.1 Building a Support Network

The Role of Social Connections

Social connections are vital for emotional and psychological resilience. Research by Dr. Julianne Holt-Lunstad at Brigham Young University found that strong social connections improve longevity, reduce stress, and enhance overall health. People with robust social networks are more likely to cope effectively with stress and bounce back from adversity.

How to Cultivate Meaningful Relationships

Cultivating meaningful relationships involves active effort and intentionality. Start by identifying people who uplift and support you. Engage in regular, meaningful interactions, whether through shared activities, conversations, or simply spending time together. Show appreciation and be present in your relationships. Building trust and mutual respect lays the foundation for a supportive network that enhances resilience.

5.2 Effective Communication Skills

Active Listening and Empathy

Active listening and empathy are key components of effective communication. Active listening involves fully concentrating, understanding, and responding thoughtfully to what others say. It shows respect and helps build deeper connections. Empathy, the ability to understand and share the feelings of others, fosters trust and strengthens bonds. Practicing these skills enhances relationships and resilience.

Assertiveness and Boundary Setting

Assertiveness involves expressing your thoughts, feelings, and needs openly and honestly while respecting others. It's crucial for maintaining healthy relationships and ensuring mutual respect. Setting boundaries helps define acceptable behaviors and protect your emotional well-being. Clear communication about boundaries prevents misunderstandings and fosters healthier interactions.

5.3 Collaborative Problem-Solving

Working Through Conflicts

Conflicts are inevitable in any relationship, but how we handle them can strengthen or weaken our bonds. Collaborative problem-solving involves working together to find mutually beneficial solutions. It requires open communication, active listening, and a willingness to understand each other's perspectives. Addressing conflicts constructively enhances trust and resilience within relationships.

Building Cooperative Strategies

Building cooperative strategies involves developing methods to work together effectively. This includes setting common goals, sharing responsibilities, and supporting each other's strengths. Effective collaboration fosters a sense of teamwork and shared purpose, which strengthens relationships and enhances collective resilience.

5.4 Supporting Others in Their Resilience Journey

Being a Source of Strength

Being a source of strength for others involves offering support, encouragement, and understanding. This can mean being a good listener, providing practical help, or simply being present during difficult times. Supporting others not only helps them build resilience but also strengthens the bond between you, creating a network of mutual support.

Encouraging Growth and Resilience in Others

Encouraging growth and resilience in others involves recognizing their strengths, providing constructive feedback, and celebrating their successes. It's about fostering an environment where people feel valued and motivated to grow. By supporting others in their resilience journey, you contribute to a positive and resilient community.

Case Studies

Case Study 1: Building a Support Network

Maria, a single mother, found herself struggling with stress and isolation. She decided to join a local support group for single parents. Through regular meetings and shared experiences, Maria built strong connections with others facing similar challenges. This network provided her with emotional support, practical advice, and a sense of belonging. As a result, Maria felt more resilient and better equipped to handle life's challenges.

Case Study 2: Effective Communication and Collaborative Problem-Solving

John and Lisa, a married couple, often found themselves arguing over household responsibilities. They decided to attend a workshop on effective communication and collaborative problem-solving. By learning to actively listen and express their needs assertively, they were able to address their conflicts constructively. They developed a system for sharing responsibilities and supporting each other's goals, which strengthened their relationship and resilience.

Conclusion

Strengthening relationships is crucial for building resilience. By building a support network, developing effective communication skills, engaging in collaborative problem-solving, and supporting others, we create a foundation for enduring connections. These relationships provide us with the support, encouragement, and sense of belonging needed to navigate life's challenges. Investing in our relationships not only enhances our resilience but also fosters a resilient community.

Resources

1. **Books**

   - "The Gifts of Imperfection" by Brené Brown

   - "Nonviolent Communication: A Language of Life" by Marshall B. Rosenberg

2. **Articles**

   - "The Importance of Social Connections" – American Psychological Association

   - "Effective Communication Strategies" – Mayo Clinic

3. **Websites**

   - Psychology Today (www.psychologytoday.com)

   - Greater Good Science Center (www.greatergood.berkeley.edu)

4. **Apps**

○ Calm (for mindfulness and meditation)

○ Relationship Booster (for relationship building exercises)

CHAPTER 6

THRIVING IN LIFE

"The greatest glory in living lies not in never falling, but in rising every time we fall." – Nelson Mandela

Introduction

Thriving in life goes beyond merely surviving challenges; it's about flourishing despite them. This chapter explores how embracing change, finding purpose, sustaining long-term resilience, and celebrating progress can lead to a fulfilling and resilient life. We'll delve into scientific research, share compelling case studies, and provide actionable insights to help you thrive in every aspect of your life.

6.1 Embracing Change and Uncertainty

Adaptability and Flexibility

Adaptability and flexibility are crucial traits for thriving in an ever-changing world. Dr. Carol Dweck's research on mindset demonstrates that those with a growth mindset—believing that abilities and intelligence can be developed—are more likely to adapt to change and view challenges as opportunities for growth. Embracing change with a positive attitude and a willingness to learn fosters resilience and personal growth.

Thriving Amidst Change

Adapting to change involves maintaining a positive outlook and being open to new experiences. A study by the American Psychological Association found that people who view change as a chance to learn and grow report higher levels of life satisfaction and well-being. Embracing change, rather than resisting it, allows us to thrive and make the most of new opportunities.

6.2 Finding Purpose and Meaning

The Importance of Life Purpose

Having a clear sense of purpose and meaning in life significantly enhances resilience. Dr. Victor Frankl, a renowned psychiatrist and Holocaust survivor, emphasized the importance of finding meaning in life. His work, detailed in "Man's Search for Meaning," shows that a sense of purpose can provide strength and motivation to overcome even the most severe adversities.

Techniques to Discover and Pursue Your Passion

Discovering your passion involves self-reflection and exploration. Consider what activities make you feel fulfilled and energized. Setting aside time for hobbies, volunteering, or pursuing new interests can help you uncover your passions. Once identified, setting goals and creating a plan to integrate your passions into your daily life can lead to a more meaningful and satisfying existence.

6.3 Sustaining Long-Term Resilience

Building Long-Term Resilience Strategies

Long-term resilience requires continuous effort and self-awareness. Strategies include developing a supportive social network, maintaining physical health, and engaging in regular self-care practices. Dr. Ann Masten, a leading resilience researcher, describes resilience as "ordinary magic," highlighting that everyday actions and attitudes can build lasting resilience.

Continuous Self-Improvement

Commitment to lifelong learning and personal growth is essential for sustained resilience. This involves setting aside time for self-reflection, seeking feedback, and embracing challenges as learning opportunities. Engaging in regular self-improvement activities, such as reading, taking courses, or learning new skills, helps maintain a resilient and adaptable mindset.

6.4 Celebrating Progress and Success

Reflecting on Your Journey

Taking time to reflect on your achievements and progress is crucial for maintaining motivation and resilience. Regular reflection allows you to acknowledge your growth, understand your strengths, and identify areas for improvement. Journaling, mindfulness, or discussing your experiences with a trusted friend can facilitate this reflection process.

The Power of Celebration and Recognition

Celebrating your successes, no matter how small, reinforces positive behavior and boosts morale. Recognition can come from within, through self-appreciation, or from others, through praise and acknowledgment. Celebrating milestones and achievements fosters a sense of accomplishment and encourages continued effort and perseverance.

Case Studies

Case Study 1: Embracing Change and Finding Purpose

Jessica, a mid-career professional, faced unexpected job loss due to company restructuring. Instead of seeing this as a setback, she viewed it as an opportunity to pursue her passion for environmental conservation. Jessica enrolled in courses, volunteered at local environmental organizations, and eventually secured a fulfilling job in her new field. By embracing change and finding purpose, Jessica not only adapted but thrived.

Case Study 2: Sustaining Long-Term Resilience and Celebrating Progress

Michael, a college student, struggled with anxiety and academic pressure. He developed a routine that included regular exercise, mindfulness practices, and setting achievable goals. Michael also kept a journal to track his progress and reflect on his journey. Celebrating small victories, like completing assignments on time or improving his grades, helped him stay motivated and resilient throughout his academic career.

Conclusion

Thriving in life involves embracing change, finding purpose, sustaining long-term resilience, and celebrating progress. By adopting a growth mindset, discovering and pursuing your passions, and maintaining continuous self-improvement, you can build a fulfilling and resilient life. Reflecting on and celebrating your achievements further reinforces positive behaviors and encourages ongoing growth. These practices not only enhance your personal resilience but also contribute to a thriving and fulfilling life.

Resources

1. **Books**

- ○ "Man's Search for Meaning" by Viktor E. Frankl

- ○ "Mindset: The New Psychology of Success" by Carol S. Dweck

2. **Articles**

- ○ "The Benefits of Embracing Change" – Harvard Business Review

- ○ "The Power of Purpose" – Psychology Today

3. **Websites**

- ○ Positive Psychology (www.positivepsychology.com)

- ○ Greater Good Science Center (www.greatergood.berkeley.edu)

4. **Apps**

- ○ Headspace (for mindfulness and meditation)

- ○ Habitica (for building and tracking habits)

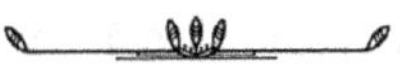

CONCLUSION

"Resilience is the capacity to recover quickly from diffi-culties; it is a measure of how effectively we can adapt to challenges and changes." – Unknown

As we come to the end of "The Resilient Mindset," it's clear that resilience is not just a trait but a journey of continuous growth and adaptation. This book has guided you through the essential components of building and maintaining resilience, providing practical strategies, scientific insights, and real-life examples to support your journey.

Reflecting on Your Resilience Journey

Throughout this book, we've explored various facets of resilience—from understanding its core concepts and building a solid foundation to overcoming adversity and cultivating positive habits. Each chapter has offered valuable tools and insights to help you navigate life's challenges and embrace opportunities for growth. Reflecting on what you've learned can help solidify these principles and integrate them into your daily life.

Applying What You've Learned

Resilience is an ongoing process that requires commitment and practice. As you apply the strategies and insights from this book, remember that setbacks are a natural part of the journey. Embrace them as opportunities for learning and growth. Regularly revisit the tools and techniques discussed in each chapter, and adjust them as needed to fit your evolving circumstances.

Embracing Continuous Improvement

One of the key themes of this book is the importance of continuous self-improvement. Building resilience is not a one-time effort but a lifelong endeavor. By remaining open to learning, setting new goals, and seeking support, you can continue to strengthen your resilience and enhance your overall well-being. Celebrate your progress and acknowledge your achievements, no matter how small they may seem.

Strengthening Your Relationships

The connections you build with others play a crucial role in your resilience. By nurturing these relationships, practicing effective communication, and supporting those around you, you create a network of mutual support that strengthens your ability to handle life's challenges. Remember that resilience is as much about your relationships with others as it is about your personal mindset.

Looking Forward

As you move forward, keep in mind that resilience is not about avoiding difficulties but about developing the capacity to face them with strength and adaptability. By embracing change, finding purpose, sustaining resilience, and celebrating your journey, you set yourself up for a life of fulfillment and success.

This book has provided a roadmap for developing a resilient mindset, but the journey is uniquely yours. Embrace the process, stay committed to growth, and approach each challenge with confidence and optimism. The resilience you build will not only help you thrive in your own life but will also inspire and support those around you.

Thank you for joining me on this journey to discover and strengthen your resilient mindset. May you continue to grow, adapt, and thrive in every aspect of your life.

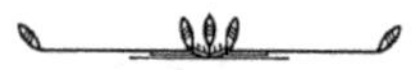